SIT, STRETCH, AND STRENGTHEN

Improve Balance, Flexibility, and Strength From Your Chair in 15 Minutes a Day
A 14-Day Program

JORDAN FRANK

Printed Worldwide
First Printing 2023
First Edition 2023

10 9 8 7 6 5 4 3 2 1

SIT, STRETCH,
AND STRENGTHEN

Table of Contents

INTRODUCTION

Exercise is vital to maintaining good physical and mental health, especially for seniors. Regular physical activity not only helps to keep us in shape, but it also helps to improve our quality of life.

As we age, we naturally start to lose muscle mass and bone density. However, regular exercise can help to slow down this process. Weight-bearing exercises can help to strengthen bones and muscles, reducing the risk of falls and fractures. It is also effective in building and maintaining muscle mass.

Physical activity is good for the heart and can help to lower the risk of heart disease, stroke, and other cardiovascular conditions. Regular exercise can help to lower blood pressure and cholesterol levels, improving overall heart health.

Regular physical activity has also been linked to improved cognitive function and a reduced risk of dementia and Alzheimer's disease.

In short, regular exercise can not only help you live a longer life, it can also help you live a fuller one. You'll see these benefits immediately. Even when you can't see the impact that your workouts are having on your heart health, you'll likely notice a significant boost in your mood.

That's because exercise releases endorphins, the "feel-good" hormones that can improve our mood and reduce stress and anxiety.

Regular exercise can also have a positive impact on sleep quality. Physical activity can help to reduce the time it takes to fall asleep, improve the depth of sleep, and reduce nighttime wakefulness.

Finally, regular exercise can help us maintain our independence and mobility. By staying active and mobile, we can reduce their risk of falls and injuries and continue to enjoy our favorite activities. Exercise can also help to improve things like balance and flexibility, leading to better overall mobility and quality of life.

By being active, you will make it easier for your body to do the things you love most. Whether that's spending time with the grandkids or hitting the links, exercise makes life much more enjoyable. Longevity is important - but it's also important to think about how you fill those extra years. Exercise checks off both boxes by extending your lifespan and making that life more meaningful. What's not to love?

However, staying active can be challenging for us older folks who may no longer have the mobility we once had. You might not be sure what kind of exercises to do or be worried that you no longer have the stamina or endurance to do the exercises you might have enjoyed in the past.

The good news is that there is no one-size-fits-all approach to exercise. You don't have to train for a marathon or bench press 300 pounds in order to stay healthy. Believe it or not, you don't even have to get out of your seat.

Chair exercises are one way to overcome the many barriers to starting a new exercise so you can stay physically fit your entire life. But what are chair exercises?

Put simply, they are seated exercises designed to help you stay active and healthy. Chair exercises don't require any equipment, and they can be done right in your living room or bedroom. They're especially beneficial for seniors who may have mobility issues or difficulty standing for long periods.

The best part? Chair exercises are easy to modify to fit your fitness level, so you can start wherever you're comfortable and work your way up. In this book, we'll give you a primer on some basic exercises you can do, but we'll also give you some tips on how to scale up the exercises as they become easier and you improve your fitness levels.

One of the most significant benefits of chair exercises is that they can help improve balance and stability. Both strength training and cardiovascular training are important types of exercises you need to include as part of your fitness routine, and chair exercises really check off both boxes.

These chair exercises are perfectly suited for those of us with partial or limited mobility. As we age, our balance can become compromised, which can lead to falls and injuries. Chair exercises are a gentle way to build up core strength, which can help improve balance over time. They can help strengthen your lower body muscles, which can reduce your risk of falling.

They can help improve flexibility and range of motion. Our joints can become stiff and immobile as we get older, making it challenging to perform daily activities. Chair exercises can help loosen up your joints and increase your flexibility, making it easier to do things like reaching overhead or bending down to pick something up.

Chair exercises can help increase blood flow to your muscles, which can help reduce aches and pains, and keep your muscles feeling loose and limber.

Last but not least, these chair exercises can improve your mood and mental health. Exercise is a proven mood-booster, and chair exercises are no exception. Physical activity can help reduce stress, anxiety, and depression, and it can increase feelings of happiness and well-being. Plus, when you feel good physically, it can have a positive impact on your mental health, too.

So what do you think? Are you ready to start breaking a sweat and getting your fitness back?

As someone who is incredibly passionate about fitness and loves learning new exercises of all kinds, I'm excited to tell you more about the best chair exercises you can do (and how to do them safely and effectively). I've worked with seniors for years, and nothing makes me happier than helping people get their mobility and lust for life back.

Doing these chair exercises is one of the best ways to live a happier, healthier, and more fulfilled life. Chances are, you'll notice an improvement almost right away!

In this book, I'll walk you through a basic 14-day workout you can do (all from your chair, and all from the comfort of your own home). I'll give you warm-up and cool-down instructions as well as modifications you can do for each of the 14 days. Of course, as I promised earlier, I'll also give you some advice on how to scale up these exercises to a higher intensity if you find that they're getting too easy.

Before I dive into the nitty-gritty of this book, I do need to get a piece of housekeeping out of the way. I am not a doctor, nor should my advice that is given in this book be taken as any type of medical advice. If you're not sure whether you can do these chair exercises safely, or if you have any underlying medical condition, please talk to your doctor first to get cleared for exercise. I don't want anyone getting hurt on my watch!

With that said, these are some safe and effective chair exercises that you should have no problem doing, even if it's been years (or perhaps an entire lifetime!) since you worked out.

So grab some water, grab a towel, and take a seat. It's time to get started!

Chapter One

A Safety Check Before You Begin

Getting older doesn't mean you have to give up physical activity. In fact, it's more important than ever that seniors maintain an active lifestyle to help prevent chronic diseases, boost mood, and stay independent.

Chair exercises are a great way to stay fit and healthy without risking injury or overexertion. Moreover, chair exercises can be done at home, making it easy to fit them into your daily routine.

There are a few things to keep in mind before you begin.

First, know that chair exercises are a great supplement or solution for any workout routine, but they don't have to be the only exercises you do. The Centers for Disease Control and Prevention recommends that adults who are 65 years of age or older get at least 150 minutes per week of moderate-intensity exercise.

These chair exercises fit the bill for most people. However, if you have a chronic health condition or have limited mobility, you may find that you need to modify these recommendations - and that's ok! Always talk to your doctor if you have any concerns about your exercise plan.

Below, I'll walk you through some other things to keep in mind as you embark on your fitness journey.

Safety Tips Before Getting Started

Staying active is vital to maintaining good health and quality of life. Chair exercises offer a great way to stay active and improve flexibility, endurance, and balance.

However, it's important to take certain safety measures before embarking on any new exercise program. So if you're ready to stay fit while sitting, here are some safety tips to keep in mind!

Consider Your Restrictions

When embarking on any new fitness routine, you've got to consider your restrictions and abilities to ensure that you don't cause more harm than good.

You should be aware of any physical conditions or limitations that may prevent you from doing certain exercises.

For example, if you have joint pain, you should avoid exercises that put stress on your joints. If you have balance issues, you should avoid exercises that require you to stand up. Knowing your limitations will help you design a workout routine that's safe and effective for your needs.

What Are Your Goals?

Setting goals in chair exercises for seniors is an excellent way to track progress and stay motivated. Make sure to manage your expectations and don't get too discouraged if you don't see results immediately. It's essential to understand that chair exercises are not a magic cure but require patience, commitment, and dedication to show positive results.

Your goals can be as complex or as simple as you'd like. I always recommend that people set SMART goals - goals that are Specific, Measurable, Actionable, Relevant, and Time-Based. It's okay to set lofty goals, but try to set some mini-goals within those that you can take small bites out of as you progress on your journey. This will help prevent you from becoming overwhelmed when you don't see progress right away.

Whatever your goals end up being, write them down and post them wherever you'll see them often - such as on your bathroom mirror or on a cupboard door in your kitchen.

Start Slowly and Build Up Gradually

Understand that starting slowly is not a sign of weakness or a lack of motivation. Everyone has to start somewhere, and not pushing yourself beyond your limits is an act of self-care. The body needs time to adjust to new stimuli, and overdoing it can cause injuries and setbacks.

Taking your time will help you to prevent burnout, stay motivated, and notice the small improvements along the way.

Come Up With a Routine

Starting slow helps you determine your physical capabilities and limits.

Consistency is key when it comes to exercise, and seniors should strive to exercise regularly. Creating a routine that works with your schedule will make it easier to stick to it. You can also invite a friend or family member to join you to make the routine more fun and enjoyable.

Use Proper Technique

Before you start the chair exercise, make sure the chair is stable and secure. Sit comfortably with your feet firmly placed on the ground and your back straight. When your back is straight, you allow the blood to flow properly, and you reduce the risk of straining your neck or back. Avoid slouching or leaning forward to prevent straining your muscles.

Start slowly and ease into the exercises. Avoid rushing into an intense workout, as this can increase the risk of injury. The warm-ups provided will help limber up stiff muscles and build strength gradually.

Breathing is an essential element of any physical activity. Make sure you are breathing deeply and steadily during your chair workout. Take a deep breath in through your nose and exhale slowly through your mouth. Proper breathing will help you maintain focus and reduce the risk of dizziness or fainting.

Give Yourself Time for Recovery

Giving your body time to recover and repair is crucial for avoiding injuries and burnout. You can do some light stretching or relaxation exercises on your rest days or simply take a break and enjoy a good book or a movie.

Remember to be patient with yourself and celebrate your small victories. Maybe you can lift your leg a bit higher than yesterday or do one more Overhead Press. These may seem like minor achievements, but they add up over time and contribute to your overall well-being.

Talk to a Doctor

Before you start any new exercise routine, it's important to talk to your doctor, especially if you have any recent injuries or medical conditions.

Listen to Your Body

When starting any new exercise routine, it's important to listen to your body. Pain is a signal that something is wrong and if ignored, it could lead to further injury or setbacks.

Body awareness is key when it comes to exercise – pay attention to how you feel during and after workouts. If something doesn't feel right, don't push through it. Take a break or modify the exercise to make it more comfortable for your body.

Be Flexible

One of the essential things to keep in mind when starting chair exercises is to be flexible. This means being open to change and adjusting your routine to fit your needs. It's crucial to listen to your body and gradually increase the duration and intensity of your exercise routine without pushing yourself too hard.

If you experience pain or discomfort while exercising, take a break and stretch it out.

When starting chair exercises, it's essential to do what feels comfortable for your body. If a particular exercise feels too challenging, modify it or skip it altogether. There's no need to force yourself to do something that doesn't feel right. You should feel energized and invigorated after exercising, not exhausted and sore.

A good rule of thumb is to do exercises that challenge you but don't push you beyond your limits.

Monitor Your Progress

One of the most effective ways to monitor progress when starting with chair exercises is to keep a record of what you're doing. Record the date, the exercises you did, how many reps you managed to complete, and for how long. Keep track of any pain points, and what you found challenging. This way, you can examine the progress you've made over weeks, months, or years.

The most rewarding thing about tracking your progress with chair exercises is the progress you can see! Celebrate small milestones with rewards, such as indulging in a treat or getting a new book. These small, consistent rewards can help to cultivate happiness and enjoyment along with the journey of chair exercises, making it easier for you to develop regular, consistent exercise habits.

Making the Most of Your Chair Exercises

Take a look at these Pro Tips for Success

Be Sure to Warm Up and Cool Down

Warm-up and cool-down are essential components of any exercise routine, whether you're doing chair exercises or anything else.

Before you jump into any physical activity, it's important to prep your body. Warming up gradually raises your heart rate, loosens up your muscles and joints, and increases blood flow to the areas you'll be working on. This helps prevent injury and ensures that your body is ready to handle the movements you'll be doing.

And once you've finished your chair exercises, it's important to take some time to cool down. Cooling down involves gradually slowing down your heart rate and bringing your body back to a resting state. Doing so can help prevent dizziness, muscle soreness, and injury.

At the end of the day, warming up and cooling down are simple but important steps that can help you get the most out of your chair exercises. So take your time, listen to your body, and never skip these important steps. Your muscles and joints will thank you!

Maintain Proper Form

Sit up straight with your feet flat on the floor. Relax your shoulders. Pay close attention to the instructions given with each exercise so that you can make the most of each and every moment.

Pace yourself

Pacing is important, too. Make sure you move at a comfortable pace when doing chair exercises. Going too fast or too slow can affect the effectiveness of your workout. If you go too fast, you may miss the proper form, and if you go too slow, you may not get your heart rate up enough to experience the benefits of cardio exercise.

Stay Hydrated

Dehydration can cause dizziness, fatigue, and muscle cramps, leading to an ineffective workout. Consider sipping on water throughout the day and having a glass of water nearby during your chair exercises.

Eat Right

A piece of fruit or a handful of nuts can be a great pre-workout snack. Fueling your body with the right foods after your workout can help your muscles recover and rebuild. Consider a protein-rich snack, such as Greek yogurt, to give your body the necessary nutrients it needs to heal and recover.

Take Breaks

Taking breaks allows your body to rest and recover before you start your next exercise. You should take a break of around 30 seconds to 1 minute in between exercises.

Pushing Through Pain? NOPE

It's common to think that if something hurts during exercise, it means you're working hard and making progress. However, this is not always the case. Pain during exercise can actually be a sign that something is wrong.

If you experience pain during chair exercises, it's important to take a step back and evaluate what might be causing it.

This may involve seeking advice from a healthcare professional or consulting with a personal trainer or fitness instructor.

Getting Enough Sleep

Starting a new exercise routine can be challenging, especially when it comes to staying motivated. Lack of sleep can affect energy levels and motivation, making it harder to get through a workout. It can also make us more prone to injuries as we may not be as alert and focused as we should be. Getting enough sleep can help boost our energy levels and motivation, making it easier to stick to a new exercise routine.

Without enough sleep, we may not be giving our muscles enough time to recover properly, which can lead to injuries and setbacks in our exercise routine.

Many chair exercises require balance and coordination. Lack of sleep can affect our balance and coordination, making it harder to perform exercises properly and increasing the risk of falls. Getting enough sleep can help improve balance and coordination, making it easier and safer to perform chair exercises.

Set a Realistic Schedule For Yourself

Don't try to push yourself too hard, especially in the beginning. Listen to your body. You might have days where you're feeling tired or sore, and that's okay. It's important to rest and take care of yourself when you need it.

Find a Friend to Exercise With You

Another thing that can help is finding a friend or group with whom to exercise. It's much easier to stay committed to something when you have others relying on you. Plus, it can be more fun to exercise with others, and you'll be more likely to stick to your routine if you enjoy the company.

Celebrate Yourself

Celebrate your progress! It can be helpful to write down your goals and track your progress, so you can see how far you've come from where you started.

When to Stop Doing These Exercises

If you experience pain or discomfort while doing any exercise, it's time to modify or stop doing them. Always listen to your body, and talk to your healthcare provider before starting any new exercise program.

Chapter Two

How to Use This Book

Are you chomping at the bit, ready to dive into your new exercise routine? Not so fast! First, let me give you a primer on how to use this book and what exactly you'll need to get started.

The first step is to get familiar with the book. The book should have everything you need to get started (e.g., instructions, illustrations, and modifications). Review the table of contents, read the introduction, and these opening chapters. The more acquainted you are with the book, the more comfortable you'll be while exercising.

Next up, follow the progression plan provided in the book. In other words, start at the beginning of the book and work your way through the exercises. Don't jump around or skip ahead; this will help you build a good foundation and avoid injury. Also, take your time. Don't rush through the exercises. Practice each movement until you feel confident, comfortable, and correct.

As you work through the book, pay close attention to your form, especially when it comes to posture, breathing, and alignment. Don't be afraid to ask for help from a qualified fitness instructor or healthcare professional if you need it.

Of course, you should modify it as needed. Not every exercise will be suitable for everyone. If an exercise doesn't feel right, skip it and try it again in a few weeks. Listen to your body, and modify the exercises as needed. Some exercises might need to be simplified, while others might need to be made more challenging. The book should provide modifications for each exercise, so use them accordingly.

Finally, set goals and track your progress. Start by setting achievable goals for yourself. For example, set a goal of exercising for ten minutes every day. Then, track your progress to see how you're doing. Keep notes at the end of each day on the pages provided. Celebrate your progress along the way, and don't forget to have fun!

What You Will Need

The right chair is the anchor of your chair exercise routine. Make sure the chair is comfortable, stable, and supportive enough to help you through various movements without sacrificing safety. Pick a chair that has a sturdy backrest that can support your entire upper torso comfortably, armrests for added support, and a cushion that can offer you the right level of comfort without being too soft or unstable.

How to Dress for These Exercises

When it comes to chair exercises, comfort is key. You want to wear clothing that allows for ease of movement and doesn't restrict you in any way. Opt for loose-fitting clothing made from soft, breathable fabrics. This could be anything from a pair of yoga pants and a T-shirt to a tracksuit or a comfortable sweatshirt.

While you may not be doing high-impact aerobics, it's still important to wear shoes that provide adequate support and stability. Your shoes should fit well and have a non-slip sole to prevent any accidents. Athletic shoes or sneakers are a good choice. Avoid footwear with high heels, as they can throw off your balance and put added stress on your joints.

One of the benefits of chair exercises is that you can do them from the comfort of your own home. This means you don't have to worry about being too cold or too hot. However, as your body warms up during your workout, you may find that you start to feel uncomfortable in what you're wearing.

That's why it's a good idea to dress in layers. You can start with a lightweight long-sleeved shirt or sweatshirt and add or remove layers as needed.

While you may want to add a little bling to your workout attire, it's important to be mindful of the jewelry you wear during chair exercises. Necklaces and bracelets can get caught on the arms or backrest of the chair, causing pain or injury. Earrings can also be a distraction or get tangled in your hair. If you do decide to wear jewelry, keep it simple and avoid anything that dangles or swings.

While not the most exciting topic, choosing the right undergarments can make all the difference during your chair workout. You want to make sure that your bra provides adequate support without being too tight or uncomfortable. For men, a comfortable pair of boxer shorts or briefs is ideal. Whatever you choose, make sure it's something that won't distract you or make you feel self-conscious during your workout.

Making Modifications

Chair exercises can be modified to suit your fitness level, physical abilities, and health conditions. Never be afraid to use smaller movements or to do fewer reps. Start slow and build up from there. As I said earlier, it's ok to skip an exercise if it doesn't feel right for you.

How to Progress as Your Strength Builds

By starting at a comfortable level, it is easier to progress gradually to more challenging exercises. Remember, consistency is key, so aim to do chair exercises for at least 10-15 minutes every day.

Once you gain an adequate level of strength and endurance, you can increase the number of repetitions you do for each exercise.

The more repetitions you do, the more effort you will need to apply to the exercise, and the more benefits you will receive from it. Also, by increasing your repetitions gradually, you lessen your chances of overexerting and injuring yourself.

As you feel ready to progress, you can add weights to your hands or wrists to strengthen your upper body. Weights should be added slowly and in small increments, as this kind of exercise can place a strain on your muscles.

Ready to get started? In the next chapter, we'll take a look at our 14 day plan for chair exercises you can easily do at home to get in shape. Let's go!

Chapter 3

14 Rotating 15 Minute Workouts

These exercises can even be done from your living room, making them an excellent option for those who can't leave their homes.

Below, you'll find a fourteen-day plan that works every part of your body over the course of two weeks. You'll rotate between arm, leg, core, full-body, and mobility days to make the most of your exercise routine while also facilitating time for rest and recovery.

Almost all of these exercises are meant to be done with just one piece of equipment - a chair! However, you can up the ante and add gear like dumbbells, kettlebells, or resistance bands if you want to make the workouts more challenging.

In addition to giving you a step-by-step breakdown on what to do each day for each exercise, I also have a built-in warm up and cool down. I've even included notes on how to progressively make the day's workout more challenging, so you can repeat these exercises and still benefit even as you progress in your fitness.

You only need about 15 minutes a day to do these exercises. With five exercises per day, plus a warm-up and cool-down, you can break those 15 minutes up however you'd like. Just make sure you don't skip the warm-up or the cool-down - these are important.

Finally, I've also added a section for notes after each day's workout. Here, you can note what went well and what didn't - so you're prepared to move on with the next set of exercises.

Ready to get started? Here's my fourteen-day guide to chair exercises to help you sit, stretch, and strengthen every part of your body.

As you progress in difficulty, remember to listen to your body and start slowly. Always prioritize proper form over quantity or intensity

Day 1

Arm Workout

This workout focuses on the arms' major muscles while preventing any risk of injury. With regular practice, you can tone your arms to stay strong and perform daily activities without struggling.

Warm Up

Start by rolling your shoulders forward and backward for ten repetitions. Then, with your arms at your side, lift your shoulders up and then down for ten repetitions. To activate the triceps in your arms, extend your arms straight overhead and then bend your elbows with forearms behind your head.

Repeat this movement for ten repetitions. Afterward, shake out your arms and get ready for the exercises.

The Exercises

Shoulder Press

You can do this exercise without weights, or you can add a small weight (around 1-2 lbs., a can of soup or a water bottle will work nicely).

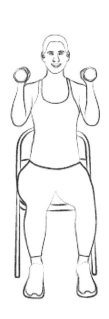 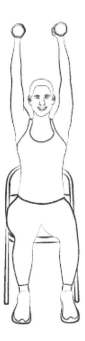

Sit up straight with feet flat on the ground and hold your weights (or no weights) in each hand. Bring your arms up so that the weights or your hands are at shoulder height and your elbows are at your sides. Inhale and lift the weights up towards the ceiling until the arms are almost straight.

Hold the weights here for 2-3 seconds before <u>slowly</u> lowering the arms back to shoulder height on a slow exhale.

REPS: 10

SETS: Start with 2

*When doing a shoulder press, imagine you're squeezing shoulder blades together as you lift and release. Keep a neutral spine alignment with the chest lifted and avoid shrugging your shoulders or letting them hunch forward as you lift and lower your arms.

As you lower the weights, maintain control so your elbows don't drop too far below shoulder height, or you will lose the strength-building benefits.

How to Progress in Difficulty:

- Increase reps to 15

- Increase sets to 3 with a minute rest in between. Do this gradually, adding a little bit each time

- Try holding the weight at the top for 3 seconds before lowering arms

2. Overhead Press

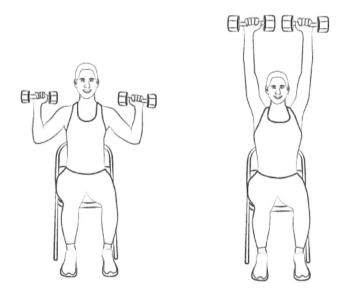

To start, sit with your back straight, and feet flat on the ground. Hold a light weight in each hand with palms facing forward.

Bend your elbows and raise your arms to shoulder level, with the elbows bent at a 90-degree angle.

Slowly straighten your arms, lifting the weights towards the ceiling, and take a deep breath. Bring the weights back down to shoulder level and exhale.

REPS: 10 (you may need to work up to this-that's OK!)

SETS: start with 1

How to Progress in Difficulty:

- Increase reps to 15 in each set
- Increase sets to 3- gradually
- Increase weight

3. Front Shoulder Raises

To start, sit comfortably with your feet flat on the ground and your back straight.

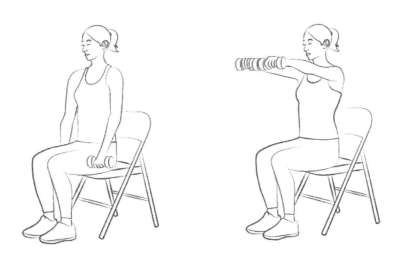

Hold a weight in each hand with your palms facing down and your arms extended down. (Its ok to not use any weights if that feels right to start with.)

Then, slowly raise your arms in front of you, keeping them straight and parallel to the ground. Stop when your arms are about shoulder level and hold for a few seconds before slowly lowering your arms back down to starting position.

REPS: 8-10

SETS: start with 2

How to Progress in Difficulty:

- Increase reps to 15 per set
- Increase sets to 3
- Increase weight (gradually)

4. Bicep Curls

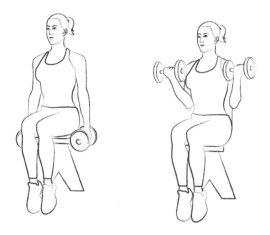

Start by sitting with your feet flat on the ground. Hold a weight in each hand, keeping your palms facing up and your elbows close to your sides. Begin with a weight that feels comfortable for you, such as 1-2 pounds.

Slowly lift the weights towards your shoulders, keeping your elbows in place by your sides. Hold the contraction for a second or two, then slowly lower the weights back down to the starting position.

REPS: 10-12

SETS: 2

It's important to focus on using your biceps to lift the weights, not your shoulders or back.

How to Progress in Difficulty:

- Increase reps to 15
- Increase sets to 3
- Increase weight, gradually
- Add a pause at the top of the movement

5. Cross Body Jabs

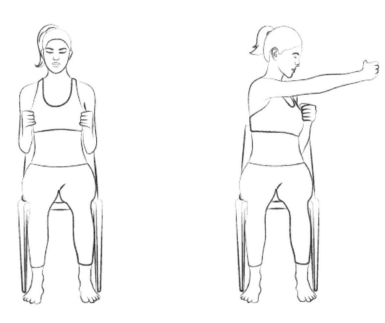

Sit up straight and place your feet hip-width apart on the floor.

Make fists in front of your chest, with your elbows bent.

Tighten your core muscles and twist your torso to the right, punching your right arm across your body towards the left. Keep your left arm stationary.

Return to the starting position and repeat on the other side, twisting your torso to the left and punching with your left arm.

Go at a speed that feels comfortable. Continue alternating punches for 30-60 seconds, or until you feel fatigued.

SETS: start with 1

How to Progress in Difficulty:

As you get more skilled with this exercise, you can make it harder by doing any of the following:

- Work your way up to 3 sets
- Increase the speed of your punches.
- Hold a small weight or resistance band in your hands.
- Add a leg lift with each punch, lifting the opposite foot off the floor as you twist.
- Try standing up and doing the exercise with or without hand weights.

Cool Down

Cooling down helps regulate blood flow and prevent muscle soreness. To cool down, perform the warm-up exercises in reverse order ten times, this time slowing the movement with each repetition.

Notes on Today's Workout

How I Felt

_____

_____

_____

_____

What I Liked

_____

_____

_____

_____

What I Would Do Differently

_____

_____

_____

_____

Day 2

Core Workout

Welcome to the second day of your chair exercise routine. In today's session, we'll be focusing on your core muscles through a range of seated exercises. You may feel intimidated by the idea of working on your core, but let me tell you, a strong core is absolutely essential to maintain a good posture, balance, and stability.

Warm Up

We'll begin with a gentle warm-up. While sitting upright in your chair, take a deep breath in, and as you exhale, draw your belly button towards your spine. Release and repeat a few times. This will help activate your core muscles and prepare them for the workout ahead.

The Exercises

Knee-to-Chest

Sit straight up in a chair with your back supported and feet flat on the floor.

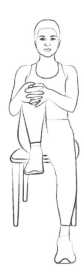

Keep your hips and shoulders aligned. Place your hands on your thighs with your palms facing down.

Lift one foot off the ground and bring your knee towards your chest, keeping your foot flat on the floor. If you need the support, you can grab the knee with your arms.

Hold this position for a few seconds, then lower your foot back down to the ground. Repeat with the other leg. As you lift your knee, exhale and engage your core muscles.

Keep your shoulders down and chest up. Aim to bring your knee as close to your chest as you can comfortably while still keeping your back straight and your other foot flat on the floor.

REPS: 5-7 on each side to start

SETS: 1-2

How to Progress in Difficulty:

- Increase reps to 10-15

- Increase sets to 3
- lift both feet off the ground at the same time and bringing your knees towards your chest

Knee extensions

Start by sitting upright in your chair with your back straight and your feet firmly planted on the ground.

Slowly extend one leg out in front of you, keeping your foot flexed and your knee in line with your hip. Flex your foot forward as if you are pushing against a wall.

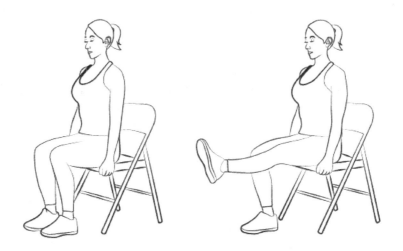

Hold the position for 2-3 seconds, then slowly lower your leg back down to the starting position.

Repeat the exercise with the other leg.

REPS: 8-12 on each leg

SETS : 1-2 to start

How to Progress in Difficulty:

To increase the difficulty of this exercise, try the following:

- Increase the number of repetitions: Gradually build up to 15-20 repetitions per leg.
- Increase sets to 3
- Add ankle weights: This will increase resistance and build strength.
- Hold a ball between your knees: This will engage your inner thigh muscles as well as your quadriceps.
- Slow down the movement: Moving more slowly will engage your muscles for longer and make the exercise more challenging.

3 Torso Turns

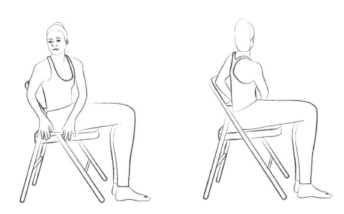

Sit straight on a chair, preferably with a backrest. Keep your feet firmly on the ground and shoulder-width apart.

Slowly twist your upper body towards the right side, taking your hands along with you.

Hold the position for a few seconds and then twist back to the starting position. Repeat the movement, twisting to the left side this time.

REPS: 10 each side

SETS: 1-2 to start

How to Progress in Difficulty:

Once you get comfortable with the basic Torso Turns, you can start adding variations to it. Here are some ideas:

- Increase reps to 15 each side
- Increase sets to 3
- Try to twist further by pushing your body a little more.
- Hold a weight in front of you while performing the torso turn. This will increase the intensity of the exercise and add more challenge to your core.

4.Modified Push-Ups

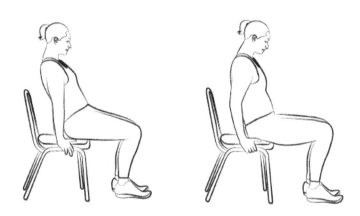

To perform a seated modified push-ups, sit on the edge of a chair and place your hands on either side of your hips, gripping the armrests.

Keeping your back straight, lift your bottom off the chair and hold it for 10 seconds.

Then, lower it back down to the chair. It's important to engage your core muscles while performing this exercise. If you find the exercise challenging, you can start by doing the movement less intensely, such as gently lifting your bottom off the chair instead of holding it or even lifting just one cheek. You will gradually work your way up to the full movement.

REPS: 8-10

SETS: 1 to start

How to Progress in Difficulty:

- Increase reps to 12-15
- Increase sets to 3
- Try lifting one leg off the ground at a time during the hold
- Increase the holding time from 10 seconds to 20 seconds

Seated Alternating Toe Touches

Sit on the edge of your chair, ideally with your feet flat on the floor and hip-width apart.

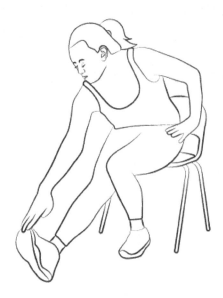

Lift your right leg off the floor and extend it forward, keeping it straight.

Reach your left hand towards your right toe, exhaling deeply as you do this. Try to touch your toe, but if you cannot reach, aim for your shin or ankle. Hold this position for a second or two, then return your arm and leg to the starting position. Repeat the same movement on your left side, alternating between your right and left leg. Remember to maintain proper form throughout the exercise, keeping your back straight, and your core engaged as you reach for your toes.

REPS: 10-12 for each leg

SETS: 1 to start

How to Progress in Difficulty:

- Increase reps to 15

- Increase sets to 3

- Hold a weighted ball or a water bottle in your hands while performing the exercise to add resistance.

- Instead of touching your toes with your opposite hand, reach with both hands for your toes, working your abdominal muscles more intensely.
- Lift both legs off the ground and reach for your toes with both hands at the same time.

Cool Down

Take a deep breath in, and as you exhale, relax your entire body. Lower your shoulders, release any tension in your neck and back. You've done a great job!

Notes on Today's Workout

How I Felt

_____

_____

_____

_____

_____

What I Liked

_____

_____

_____

_____

_____

What I Would Do Differently

_____

_____

_____

_____

_____

Day 3

Leg Day

Today, we're focusing on leg day and I am ready to lead you through some simple yet effective exercises to help strengthen and tone your lower body.

Warm Up

Start by sitting tall in your chair with your feet flat on the ground. Gently roll your shoulders back and down and take a few deep breaths. Next, begin to march your feet in place, lifting your knees as high as you comfortably can.

Do this for about 30 seconds to increase blood flow to your legs and get your heart rate up.

The Exercises

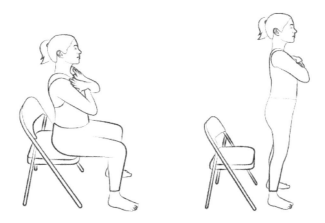

Sit/Stand

Begin by standing in front of a sturdy chair with your feet shoulder-width apart and your toes pointing forward. Slowly sit down into the chair, keeping your back straight and bending your knees.

Once you're seated, pause for a moment before standing back up, using your leg muscles to push yourself up to a standing position. If you need to, it's ok to use your arms for assistance. We will gradually work up to a point where you don't need them!

REPS: 6-8 (adjust for your abilities)

SETS: 1 to start

How to Progress in Difficulty:

- Increase reps to 15
- Increase number of sets to 3
- Hold onto a water bottle or lightweight to add resistance to the exercise.
- Lift one leg up while completing the exercise to activate more muscles and increase balance.

2. Leg Circles

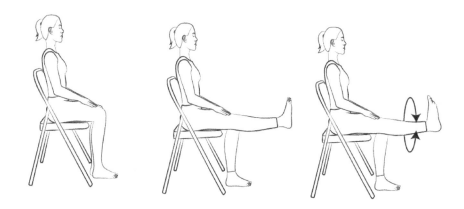

Begin by sitting upright in a chair with your back straight and your feet firmly planted on the floor. Make sure the chair is sturdy and won't move around. Place your hands on the sides of the chair for support.

Lift one leg up, so your knee is at a 90-degree angle, parallel to the floor. Keep your foot flexed for stability. Slowly rotate your leg in a circular motion, starting from your hip joint. Make sure to keep your back straight and your core engaged throughout the exercise.

Complete the circle by bringing your leg down and back to its starting position.

REPS: 8-10/leg

SETS: 1 to start

How to Progress in Difficulty:

- Increase the number of repetitions to 15 gradually
- Increase the number of sets to 3
- Add ankle weights for more resistance
- Increase the size of the circular motion
- Alternate directions, working both clockwise and counterclockwise

3. Heel Slides

Sit upright in a sturdy chair with your feet flat on the ground and your back straight.

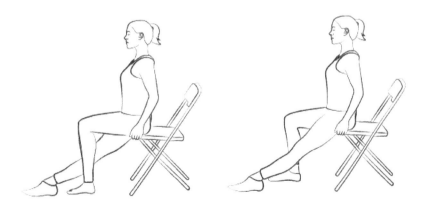

Slowly slide your right heel towards your buttocks, bending your knee as far as you comfortably can.

Hold the position for a few seconds, then slowly slide your heel back to the starting position.

Repeat on the other side, alternating between your left and right heel.

REPS: 15 per leg

SETS: start with 1

How to Progress in Difficulty:

- Work up to 3 sets
- You can make heel slides more challenging by wearing ankle weights, starting with 1 or 2 pounds and gradually increasing the weight.
- Alternate legs in a skating motion

4. Calf Raises

Sit on the edge of a sturdy chair with your feet flat on the ground.

Place your hands on your thighs or hold onto the sides of the seat.

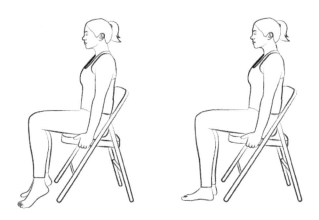

Slowly raise your heels, keeping your toes on the ground until you feel your calf muscle engaged.

Pause for 2-3 seconds, then slowly lower your heels back to the ground.

REPS: 10-12

SETS: start with one

How to Progress in Difficulty:

- Increase reps to 15-20
- Work up to 3 sets
- Hold a lightweight, like a water bottle, in each hand while doing calf raises.
- Hold the top of the calf raise for an extra few seconds before lowering your heels.

5. Glute Squeezes

First, sit on a sturdy, non-slip chair with your feet planted firmly on the ground. Keep your back straight, shoulders relaxed, and hands resting on your thighs.

Next, tighten your glutes by squeezing your buttocks muscles. Hold for a count of 5, then release slowly. There is no picture here….but YOU'VE GOT THIS!!

REPS: 5-10

SETS: 1 to start

How to Progress in Difficulty:

- Increase reps to 10-15
- Work up to 3 sets
- Increase the duration of each squeeze and release.
- Add resistance by placing a folded towel or cushion between your knees.
- Lift one foot slightly off the ground while squeezing with the opposite glute.

Notes on Today's Workout

How I Felt

_____

_____

_____

_____

What I Liked

_____

_____

_____

_____

What I Would Do Differently

_____

_____

_____

_____

Day 4

Mobility Work Day

By now, you should have improved your strength, balance, and body coordination from the previous exercises. Today, we'll focus on mobility work day which involves stretching. Stretching helps improve flexibility, mobility, and joint mobility to allow you to move with ease.

Warm Up

Sit up straight, keep your shoulders away from your ears and relax. Raise your shoulders up to your ears, and then roll them back and down. Rotate your shoulders backward for five seconds, and then forward for another five seconds.

Sitting up straight, lower your right ear to your right shoulder, hold for ten seconds, and then roll your head slowly and gently back. Repeat the same motion on the other side. Do this 5 or 6 times on each side. It should feel good!

You're ready to start the exercises!

The Exercises

Neck Turns

Start by sitting in a comfortable chair with your feet flat on the ground and hands resting on your lap.

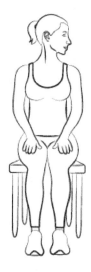 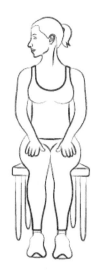

Begin by looking straight ahead and then slowly turn your head to look over your right shoulder. Hold the position for a few seconds and then return to the center.

Repeat on the left side.

REPS: 10 on each side

SETS: 1 to start

How to Progress in Difficulty:

- Increase reps to 15

- Work up to 3 sets

- Hold a small weight, such as a water bottle, with both hands and place it on your forehead. Then slowly turn your head to the right while keeping the weight in place. Hold for a few seconds and return to the center.

Shoulder Shrug

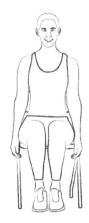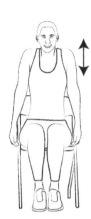

Sit on a chair with your back straight and your feet flat on the floor. Hold a weight or a water bottle (or nothing!) in each hand and let your arms hang down by your sides. Slowly lift your shoulders towards your ears while keeping your arms straight and exhaling.

Hold the tension in your shoulders for 2-3 seconds, then lower your shoulders back down while inhaling. Push shoulders down and hold for 2-3 seconds .

REPS: 10-15

SETS: 1 start

How to Progress in Difficulty:

To make this exercise more difficult:

- Work you way up to 3 sets
- Add or increase the weight of your weights
- Hold the tension in your shoulders for a longer period
- Try alternating shoulder shrugs by lifting your left shoulder up while lowering your right shoulder and vice versa

3. Side Stretch

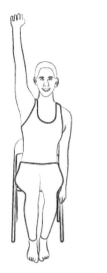 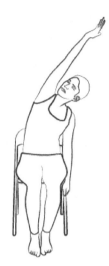

Sit in a chair with your feet flat on the ground and your hands resting on your lap. Ensure that your chest is up, your shoulders are relaxed, and your spine is straight.

Place your right hand on the side of your chair and reach upwards with your left hand to stretch your left arm up over your head and bend to the right.

Hold the stretch for 20-30 seconds, inhaling and exhaling deeply.

Bring your left hand down to rest on your lap, then repeat the stretch on the opposite side, using your left hand on the side of the chair and your right arm reaching upwards.

REPS: 5 stretches on each side

SETS: 1 to start

How to Progress in Difficulty:

- Increase the number of repetitions you do per session.

- Work your way up to 3 sets
- Gradually increase the range of motion by stretching your arms further as you bend to the side.
- Alternate the seated side stretch with standing side stretches to increase the intensity of the exercise.

4. Overhead Stretch

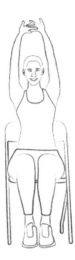

Start by sitting up straight on a sturdy chair with your feet flat on the ground. Place your hands on your thighs. Inhale and lift both arms up and above your head with your fingers interlaced. Keep your shoulders relaxed.

Exhale and slowly lower your arms behind your head, bending and stretching your elbows back as far as comfortable.

Hold the stretch for 10-30 seconds, feeling the stretch in your upper back and shoulders. Avoid straining your neck by keeping your gaze neutral.

Inhale and bring your arms back up to the starting position.

REPS: 3-5 times

SETS: 1 to start

How to Progress in Difficulty:

To progress in difficulty:

- Add a small weight, such as a water bottle, to each hand to increase resistance.
- Stretch your arms wider apart to intensify the stretch.
- Hold the stretch for longer periods, up to a minute.
- Perform the stretch with your eyes closed, focusing on deep breathing and relaxation.
- Work your way up to 3 sets

Seated Backbend

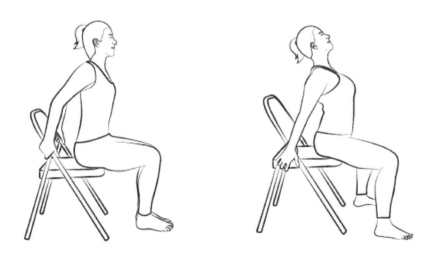

Sit forward on your chair with your feet flat on the floor and your hands on your hips or holding on to chair.

Inhale deeply and arch your back, pushing your chest forward while keeping your shoulders down.

Exhale as you return to an upright position.

REPS: 5 times

SETS: 1 to start

How to Progress in Difficulty:

☒   Increase reps to 8-10

☒   Work your way up to 3 sets

☒   Hold onto a weight or resistance band while doing the backbend.

☒   Do the exercise with your hands clasped behind your back.

☒   Hold the backbend for several seconds, then return slowly to an upright position.

Cool Down

Slowly bend forward and try to touch your toes while keeping your legs straight. Hold for ten seconds then return to the starting position.

Breathe in through your nose as deep as you can, then hold for three seconds, and breathe out through your mouth. Do this process five times.

Notes on Today's Workout

How I Felt

_____

_____

_____

_____

What I Liked

_____

_____

_____

_____

What I Would Do Differently

_____

_____

_____

_____

Day 5

Full Body Day

Welcome back! It's day 5 of our chair exercise series, and we're going to focus on the full body. If you've been following along, you're probably feeling stronger and more energized by now.

Warm Up

Sit on the chair with your back straight, feet flat on the floor and your arms at your side. Start by rotating your neck in circles, clockwise and counterclockwise.

Then, move your arms in arm circles forward and backward while keeping your back straight. Next, alternate lifting your legs up and down. Do this exercise for about 30 seconds on each side.

Finally, take a deep breath and stretch your arms up to the ceiling. We're ready to start!

The Exercises

Shoulder Press

You can do this exercise with no weights, or you can add a small weight (around 1-2 lbs – again, a can of soup or a water bottle will work nicely).

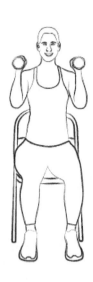
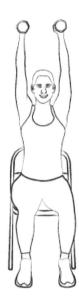

Sit up straight with feet flat on the ground, and hold a set of light weights (or no weights) in each hand. Bring your arms up so that the weights or your hands are at shoulder height and your elbows are at your sides. Inhale and lift the up towards the ceiling until the arms are almost straight.

Hold the weights here for a brief moment before **<u>slowly</u>** lowering the arms back to shoulder height on a slow exhale.

REPS: 10

SETS: Start with 2

When doing a shoulder press, imagine you're squeezing shoulder blades together as you lift and release. Keep a neutral spine alignment with the chest lifted, and avoid shrugging your shoulders or letting them hunch forward as you lift and lower your arms.

As you lower the weights, maintain control so your elbows don't drop too far below shoulder height, or you will lose the strength-building benefits.

How to Progress in Difficulty:

- Increase reps to 15
- Increase sets to 3 with a minute rest in between. Do this gradually, adding a little bit each time
- Try holding the weight at the top for 3 seconds before lowering arms

March in Place

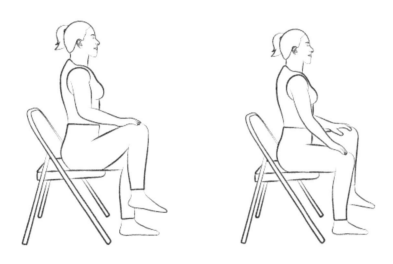

Sit up straight in your chair with your feet flat on the floor. Make sure your chair is stable and won't tip over. Keep your back straight and engage your core muscles.

Start by marching only your right leg up and down, as if you're marching in place. Keep the movement slow and controlled.

After 30 seconds, switch to your left leg and march for another 30 seconds. Repeat the cycle.

REPS: 1 30 second march on each side

SETS: start with 1

How to Progress in Difficulty:

To progress:

- Increase to 2, then 3 sets
- Try raising your knees higher
- Add ankle weights
- Introduce hand weights while marching

3. Ankle Circles

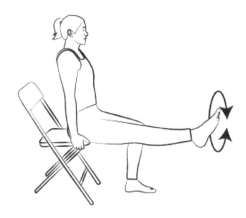

Sit on a chair with your back straight and your feet flat on the ground.

Lift your right foot off the ground and rotate just your foot clockwise for 10-15 seconds(not the whole leg).

Rotate your foot counterclockwise for 10-15 seconds.

Repeat this with your left foot.

REPS: 10-15 seconds per foot

SETS: start with 2

How to Progress in Difficulty:

- Gradually increase the time you spend on each rotation until you can do 30 seconds each way.
- Increase sets to 3
- Try the exercise with your eyes closed. This is a great way to challenge your balance and improve stability.
- Add ankle weights.

4. Knee Extensions

Start by sitting upright in your chair with your back straight and your feet firmly planted on the ground.

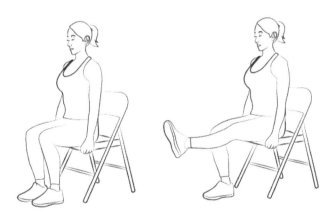

Slowly extend one leg out in front of you, keeping your foot flexed and your knee in line with your hip. Flex your foot forward as if you are pushing against a wall.

Hold the position for 2-3 seconds, then slowly lower your leg back down to the starting position.

Repeat the exercise with the other leg.

REPS: 8-12 on each leg

SETS: 1-2 to start

How to Progress in Difficulty:

To increase the difficulty of this exercise, try the following:

- Increase the number of repetitions: Gradually build up to 15-20 repetitions per leg.
- Increase sets to 3
- Add ankle weights: This will increase resistance and build strength.
- Hold a ball between your knees: This will engage your inner thigh muscles as well as your quadriceps.
- Slow down the movement: Moving more slowly will engage your muscles for longer and make the exercise more challenging.

5.Alternating Cross Body Crunch

Begin by sitting straight on a chair. Put your hands behind your head or grip the chair with both hands.

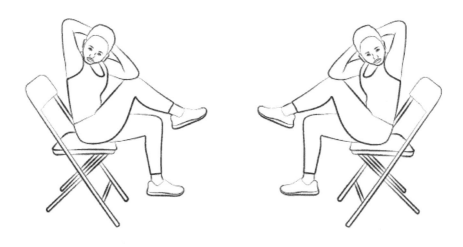

Lift your right knee and bring it towards your left elbow, twisting your torso to the right. Repeat on the other side: lift your left knee and bring it towards your right elbow while twisting to the left.

Do this in alternating fashion, as if you are pedaling a bicycle while crunching your sides.

REPS: 8-10 each side

SETS: start with 1

How to Progress in Difficulty:

⊠   Increase reps to 12-15 each side

⊠   Work up to 3 sets

⊠   Hold a water bottle in each hand while executing the crunches for added resistance.

⊠   Slow down the motion and hold each side crunch for 2-3 seconds before switching to the other side.

Cool Down

Sit with your feet flat on the ground, take a few deep breaths, and stretch your arms out. Rotate your neck, and take the time to relax your muscles. Then you can stand up and start the rest of your day feeling energized!

Notes on Today's Workout

How I Felt

_____

_____

_____

_____

What I Liked

_____

_____

_____

_____

What I Would Do Differently

_____

_____

_____

_____

Day 6

Arm Day

Are you ready for Day 6 of our Chair Exercises for Seniors? Today is all about arm day, and we have a great workout in store for you. So, let's get started!

Warm Up

Sit up straight and raise both of your arms out to the sides, keeping them at shoulder height. Then, slowly rotate them in a circular motion for about 30 seconds. Repeat this for two sets and then rest for 10 seconds. This warm-up will loosen up your muscles and prepare you for the workout.

The Exercises

Front Shoulder Raises

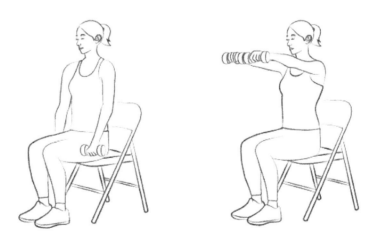

To start, sit comfortably in a chair with your feet flat on the ground and your back straight.

Hold a weight in each hand with your palms facing down and your arms extended down. (It's ok to not use any weights if that feels right to start with.)

Then, slowly raise your arms in front of you, keeping them straight and parallel to the ground. Stop when your arms are about shoulder level and hold for a few seconds before slowly lowering your arms back down to starting position.

REPS: 8-10

SETS: start with 2

How to Progress in Difficulty:

- Increase reps to 15 per set
- Increase sets to 3
- Increase weight (gradually)

Triceps Extensions

Sit on your chair with your back straight and hold a weight with both hands behind your head.

Keep your elbows close to your ears and extend your arms up to bring the dumbbell straight above your head.

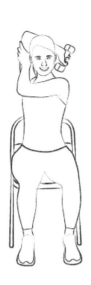 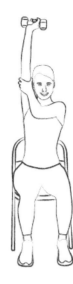

Now slowly lower the dumbbell down to the nape of your neck while keeping your elbows close to your ears.

REPS: 8-10

SETS: 2

How to Progress in Difficulty:

- Increase reps to 15
- Work your way up to 3 sets
- Gradually increase the weight

Bow String Pull-Back

Sit on a sturdy and comfortable chair. Sit up tall with your feet flat on the floor and back straight. Engage your core muscles.

Stretch your arms out straight in front of you, palms facing each other.

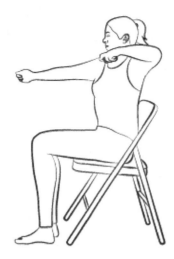

Slowly pull your right arm back as if you're pulling a bow string. As you do so, squeeze your shoulder blades together, hold for a few seconds, then release. Repeat using the left arm to pull.

Remember to breathe regularly throughout the exercise. The movement should be smooth and controlled.

REPS: 10-12

SETS: start with 2

How to Progress in Difficulty:

- Increase reps to 15
- Work your way up to 3 sets
- increase the intensity by adding weight to both hand

4. Cross Body Jabs

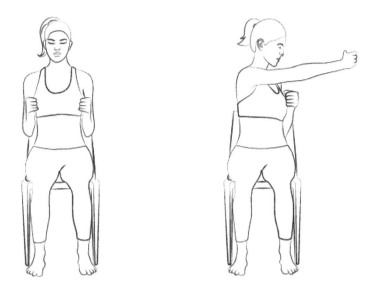

Sit up straight and place your feet hip-width apart on the floor.

Make 2 fists in front of your chest, with your elbows bent.

Tighten your core muscles and twist your torso to the right, punching your right arm across your body towards the left. Keep your left arm stationary.

Return to the starting position and repeat on the other side, twisting your torso to the left and punching with your left arm.

Continue alternating punches for 30-60 seconds, or until you feel fatigued.

REPS: 1 rep is 30-60 seconds

SETS: start with 1 set

How to Progress in Difficulty:

- Increase the length of the rep to full 60 seconds
- Work your way up to 3 sets

- Increase the speed of your punches.

- Hold a small weight or resistance band in your hands.

- Add a leg lift with each punch, lifting the opposite foot off the floor as you twist.

5. Overhead Stretch

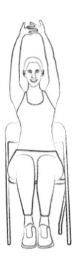

Start by sitting up straight on a sturdy chair with your feet flat on the ground. Place your hands on your thighs.

Inhale and lift both arms up and above your head. Grasp your hands together if you can.

Exhale and slowly lower your arms behind your head, bending and stretching your elbows back as far as comfortable.

Hold the stretch for 10-30 seconds, feeling the stretch in your upper back and shoulders. Avoid straining your neck by keeping your gaze neutral.

Inhale and bring your arms back up to the starting position.

REPS: 3-5 times

SETS: 1 to start

How to Progress in Difficulty:

- Add a small weight, such as a water bottle, to each hand to increase resistance.
- Stretch your arms wider apart to intensify the stretch.
- Hold the stretch for longer periods, up to a minute.
- Perform the stretch with your eyes closed, focusing on deep breathing and relaxation.
- Work your way up to 3 sets

Cool Down

Cool down with some light stretching for your arms and shoulders. Sit up straight and reach your arms out in front of you, then slowly pull them towards your body, stretching your arms and shoulders. Hold this position for 10-15 seconds and then release. Repeat this for two sets.

Notes on Today's Workout

How I Felt

_____

_____

_____

_____

_____

What I Liked

_____

_____

_____

_____

_____

What I Would Do Differently

_____

_____

_____

_____

Day 7

Core Work

Today, we're focusing on our core - the muscles that support our back, improve our posture, and aid in our daily movements. Core strength is essential to maintain a healthy and active lifestyle, especially for seniors.

Warm Up

Start by sitting upright in your chair, with your feet flat on the ground and your hands resting on your thighs.

Take a deep breath in, and as you exhale, twist your upper body to the right. Hold for a few seconds, then inhale and come back to center. Exhale, twist to the left, and hold for a few seconds. Repeat on each side.

Next, sit at the edge of your chair and lift one knee up towards your chest, placing your hands behind your thigh to assist. Hold for a few seconds, then lower your foot back to the ground. Repeat on the other side. You're ready to get started!

The Exercises

Seated Jack

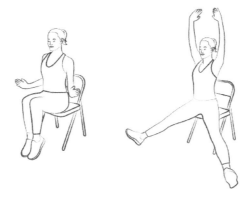

Sit up straight in your chair with your feet firmly planted on the ground.

Place your hands on the armrests of your chair and begin moving feet in and out (as if you were doing a jumping jack motion with your lower body).

As you move, bring your hands overhead and clap them together at the top of the motion.

Keep your movements controlled and steady, making sure to engage your core muscles throughout the exercise.

REPS: Continue for 30 seconds

SETS: start with 1

How to Progress in Difficulty:

- Increase rep to 60 seconds
- Work your way up to 3 sets
- Increase the speed of movements
- Hold onto a weight

2. Alternating Toe Touches

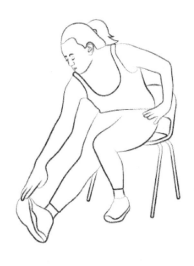

Sit on the edge of your chair, ideally with your feet flat on the floor and hip-width apart.

Lift your right leg off the floor and extend it forward, keeping it straight. Reach your left hand towards your right toe, exhaling deeply as you do this. Try to touch your toe, but if you cannot reach, aim for your shin or ankle.

Hold this position for a second or two, then return your arm and leg to the starting position. Repeat the same movement on your left side, alternating between your right and left leg. Remember to maintain proper form throughout the exercise, keeping your back straight, and your core engaged as you reach for your toes.

REPS: 10-12 for each leg

SETS: 1 to start

How to Progress in Difficulty:

- Increase reps to 15
- Increase sets to 3
- Hold a weighted ball or a water bottle in your hands while performing the exercise to add resistance.
- Instead of touching your toes with your opposite hand, reach with both hands for your toes, working your abdominal muscles more intensely.
- Lift both legs off the ground and reach for your toes with both hands at the same time.

3. Side Stretch

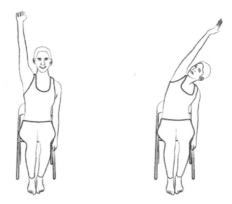

Sit in a chair with your feet flat on the ground and your hands resting on your lap. Ensure that your chest is up, your shoulders are relaxed, and your spine is straight. Place your right hand on the side of your chair and reach upwards with your left hand to stretch your left arm up over your head and bend to the right.

Hold the stretch for 20-30 seconds, inhaling and exhaling deeply.

Bring your left hand down to rest on your lap, then repeat the stretch on the opposite side, using your left hand on the side of the chair and your right arm reaching upwards.

REPS: 5 stretches on each side

SETS: 1 to start

How to Progress in Difficulty:

- Increase the number of repetitions you do per session.
- Work your way up to 3 sets
- Gradually increase the range of motion by stretching your arms further as you bend to the side.

- Alternate the seated side stretch with standing side stretches to increase the intensity of the exercise.

4. Alternating Cross Body Crunch

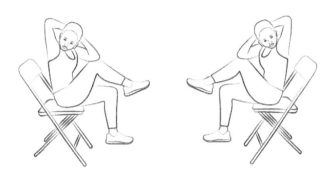

Begin by sitting straight on a chair. Put your hands behind your head or grip the chair with both hands.

Lift your right knee and bring it towards your left elbow, twisting your torso to the right. Repeat on the other side: lift your left knee and bring it towards your right elbow while twisting to the left.

Do this in alternating fashion, as if you are pedaling a bicycle while crunching your sides.

REPS: 8-10 each side

SETS: start with 1

How to Progress in Difficulty

- Increase reps to 12-15 each side
- Work up to 3 sets

- Hold a water bottle in each hand while executing the crunches for added resistance.

- Slow down the motion and hold each side crunch for 2-3 seconds before switching to the other side.

5.Seated Backbend

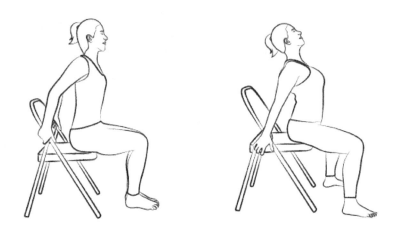

Sit forward on your chair with your feet flat on the floor and your hands on your hips.

Inhale deeply and arch your back, pushing your chest forward while keeping your shoulders down. Keep your chin up and facing forward.

Exhale as you return to an upright position.

REPS: 5 times

SETS: 1 to start

How to Progress in Difficulty:

- Increase reps to 8-10

- Work your way up to 3 sets

- Hold onto a weight or resistance band while doing the backbend.

- Do the exercise with your hands clasped behind your back.

- Hold the backbend for several seconds, then return slowly to an upright position.

Cool Down

Take a deep breath in, and as you exhale, bring your arms up towards the ceiling. Interlace your fingers and release your palms towards the ceiling. Take another deep breath in, and as you exhale, lower your arms back down to your sides. Repeat for 5 reps.

Notes on Today's Workout

How I Felt

_____

_____

_____

_____

What I Liked

_____

_____

_____

_____

What I Would Do Differently

_____

_____

_____

_____

Day 8

Leg Day

Today, we will be focusing on leg day. Our legs are vital in our daily activities, and giving them a good workout will keep them strong and healthy as we age.

Warm Up

Before we start, it's essential to do a quick warm-up. Start by sitting up straight in your chair and place your feet flat on the floor.

Slowly lift one leg, bending at the knee, and hold it for a few seconds. Then gently release it and do the same with the other leg. This exercise will help warm up your leg muscles and get them ready for more intensive movements.

The Exercises

1. Leg Circles

Begin by sitting upright in a chair with your back straight and your feet firmly planted on the floor. Make sure the chair is sturdy and won't move around. Place your hands on the sides of the chair for support.

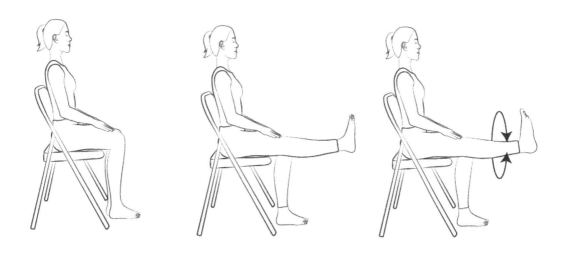

Lift one leg up, so your knee is at a 90-degree angle, parallel to the floor. Keep your foot flexed for stability.

Slowly rotate your leg in a circular motion, starting from your hip joint. Make sure to keep your back straight and your core engaged throughout the exercise.

Complete the circle by bringing your leg down and back to its starting position.

REPS: 8-10/leg

SETS: 1 to start

How to Progress in Difficulty:

- Increase the number of repetitions to 15, gradually
- Increase the number of sets to 3
- Add ankle weights for more resistance
- Increase the size of the circular motion
- Alternate directions, working both clockwise and counterclockwise

2. Toe Taps

Sit towards the front of your chair with your feet flat on the floor.

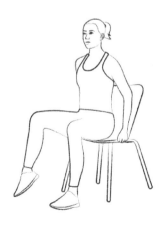

Keep your back straight and engage your core muscles. Lift your right foot off the floor and tap your toes lightly on the ground. Then, lift your left foot and tap your toes.

Continue alternating between your right and left foot, tapping your toes 30 seconds. It's important to keep your movements slow and controlled and avoid bouncing your feet off the floor.

REPS: 30 seconds

SETS: 1-2

How to Progress in Difficulty

- Increase Reps to 60 seconds
- Work your way up to 3 sets
- Try moving your feet in a faster rhythm while still maintaining control.
- Instead of tapping your toes, try tapping your heels. Alternatively, you can tap your left foot twice before alternating to the right foot. This will help to engage different muscle groups.
- Add arm raises or punches while you tap your toes. This will help to engage your upper body as well.

3. Sit/Stand

Begin by standing in front of a sturdy chair with your feet shoulder-width apart and your toes pointing forward.

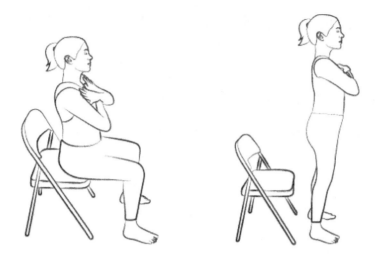

Slowly sit down into the chair, keeping your back straight and bending your knees. Once you're seated, pause for a moment before standing back up, using your leg muscles to push yourself up to a standing position. If you need to, it's ok to use your arms for assistance. We will gradually work up to a point where you don't need them!

REPS: 6-8 (adjust for your abilities)

SETS: 1 to start

How to Progress in Difficulty:

- Increase reps to 15
- Increase number of sets to 3
- Hold onto a water bottle or lightweight to add resistance to the exercise.
- Lift one leg up while completing the exercise to activate more muscles and increase balance.

4. March in Place

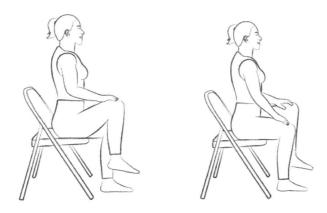

Sit up straight in your chair with your feet flat on the floor. Make sure your chair is stable and won't tip over. Keep your back straight and engage your core muscles. Start by marching only your right leg up and down, as if you're marching in place. Keep the movement slow and controlled.

After 30 seconds, switch to your left leg and march for another 30 seconds. Repeat the cycle.

REPS: One 30 second march on each side

SETS: start with one set

How to Progress in Difficulty:

To progress:

- Increase to 2, then 3 sets
- Try raising your knees higher
- Add ankles weights
- Introduce hand weights while marching

5. Calf Raises

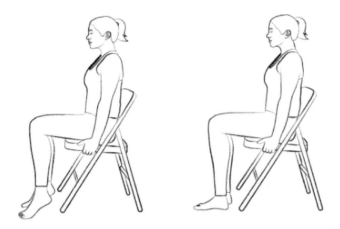

Sit on the edge of a sturdy chair with your feet flat on the ground.

Place your hands on your thighs or hold onto the sides of the seat.

Slowly raise your heels, keeping your toes on the ground until you feel your calf muscle engaged.

Pause for 2-3 seconds, then slowly lower your heels back to the ground.

REPS: 10-12

SETS: start with one

How to Progress in Difficulty:

- Increase reps to 15-20
- Work up to 3 sets
- Hold a lightweight, like a water bottle, in each hand while doing calf raises.
- Hold the top of the calf raise for an extra few seconds before lowering your heels.

Cool Down

Start by sitting up straight and take a few deep breaths. Then, lift your right leg and gently stretch it towards your chest, holding it for a few seconds. Release and do the same with your left leg.

Notes on Today's Workout

How I Felt

_____

_____

_____

_____

What I Liked

_____

_____

_____

_____

What I Would Do Differently

_____

_____

_____

_____

Day 9

Full Body Day

Today, we will be focusing on full-body workouts, which will help keep your body active and improve your overall health and fitness.

Warm Up

For today's warm-up, we will start with marching in place with the arms swinging back and forth. Then, lift your knees to your hips while swinging your arms back and forth. You should feel your heart rate increasing and your body slowly loosening up.

The Exercises

1 Shoulder Press

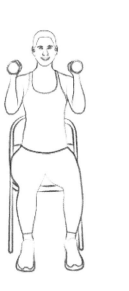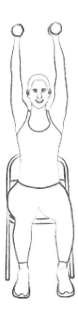

You can do this exercise with no weights, or you can add a small weight (around 1-2 lbs – again, a can of soup or a water bottle will work nicely).

Sit up straight with feet flat on the ground and hold a set of light weights (or no weights) in each hand. Bring your arms up so that the weights or your hands are at shoulder height and your elbows are at your sides. Inhale and lift the weights up towards the ceiling until the arms are almost straight.

Hold the weights here for a brief moment before **slowly** lowering the arms back to shoulder height on a slow exhale.

REPS: 10

SETS: Start with 2

When doing a shoulder press, imagine you're squeezing shoulder blades together as you lift and release. Keep a neutral spine alignment with the chest lifted and avoid shrugging your shoulders or letting them hunch forward as you lift and lower your arms.

As you lower the weights, maintain control so your elbows don't drop too far below shoulder height, or you will lose the strength-building benefits.

How to Progress in Difficulty:

- Increase reps to 15
- Increase sets to 3 with a minute rest in between. Do this gradually, adding a little bit each time
- Try holding the weight at the top for 3 seconds before lowering arms

2.Knee Extensions

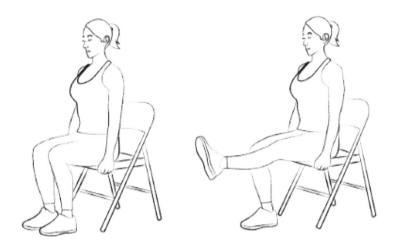

Start by sitting upright in your chair with your back straight and your feet firmly planted on the ground.

Slowly extend one leg out in front of you, keeping your foot flexed and your knee in line with your hip. Flex your foot forward as if you are pushing against a wall.

Hold the position for 2-3 seconds, then slowly lower your leg back down to the starting position.

Repeat the exercise with the other leg.

REPS: 8-12 on each leg

SETS : 1-2 to start

How to Progress in Difficulty:

To increase the difficulty of this exercise, try the following:

- Increase the number of repetitions: Gradually build up to 15-20 repetitions per leg.

- Increase sets to 3

- Add ankle weights: This will increase resistance and build strength.

- Hold a ball between your knees: This will engage your inner thigh muscles as well as your quadriceps.

- Slow down the movement: Moving more slowly will engage your muscles for longer and make the exercise more challenging.

3. Cross Body Jabs

Sit up straight and place your feet hip-width apart on the floor.

Make fists in front of your chest with your elbows bent.

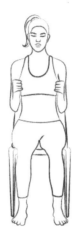 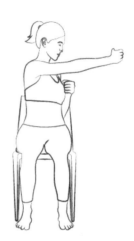

Tighten your core muscles and twist your torso to the right, punching your right arm across your body towards the left. Keep your left arm stationary.

Return to the starting position and repeat on the other side, twisting your torso to the left and punching with your left arm.

Continue alternating punches for 30-60 seconds, or until you feel fatigued.

SETS: start with 1

How to Progress in Difficulty:

As you get more skilled with this exercise, you can make it harder by doing any of the following:

- Increase the speed of your punches.
- Hold a small weight or resistance band in your hands.
- Add a leg lift with each punch, lifting the opposite foot off the floor as you twist.
- Try standing up and doing the exercise with or without hand weights.

4. Seated Jack

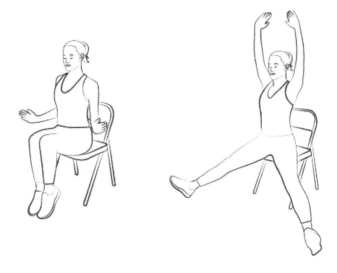

Sit up straight in your chair with your feet firmly planted on the ground.

Place your hands on the armrests of your chair and begin moving feet in and out (as if you were doing a jumping jack motion with your lower body).

As you move, bring your hands overhead and clap them together at the top of the motion.

Keep your movements controlled and steady, making sure to engage your core muscles throughout the exercise.

REPS: Continue for 30 seconds

SETS: start with 1

How to Progress in Difficulty:

- Increase rep to 60 seconds
- Work your way up to 3 sets
- Increase the speed of movements
- Hold onto a weight

5. Torso Turns

Sit straight on a chair, preferably with a backrest. Keep your feet firmly on the ground and shoulder-width apart.

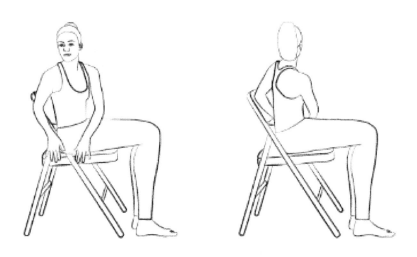

Slowly twist your upper body towards the right side, taking your hands along with you.

Hold the position for a few seconds and then twist back to the starting position. Repeat the movement, twisting to the left side this time.

REPS: 10 each side

SETS: 1-2 to start

How to Progress in Difficulty:

Once you get comfortable with the basic Seated Tummy Turn, you can start adding variations to it. Here are some ideas:

- Increase reps to 15 each side
- Increase sets to 3
- Try to twist further by pushing your body a little more.
- Hold a weight in front of you while performing the tummy twists. This will increase the intensity of the exercise and add more challenge to your core.

Cool Down

For today's cool-down, we will do some simple stretches. Sit up straight and stretch your arms up, take a deep breath, hold, then release. Stretch your arms out to each side and hold, then release. Finally, stretch your arms down, touch your toes, and hold for a few seconds.

Notes on Today's Workout

How I Felt

_____

_____

_____

_____

What I Liked

_____

_____

_____

_____

What I Would Do Differently

_____

_____

_____

_____

Day 10

Mobility Day

Today we will focus on mobility exercises that will help improve your range of motion, flexibility, and balance. As you age, mobility becomes more challenging, and these exercises will help you regain your confidence and independence.

Warm Up

Before we begin the mobility exercises, we will do a quick warm-up session to loosen up your muscles and prepare your body for the session.

Let's raise our arms above our heads and slowly move them from side to side, exhaling as we stretch. Now rotate your neck gently, looking left and right, up and down, and then shoulder rolls to loosen up those stiff joints.

Lastly, lift your legs slightly off the ground and flex your feet back and forth. Great job - now let's move on.

The Exercises

Chest Stretch

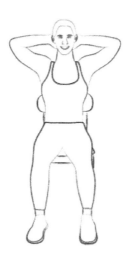

Begin by sitting comfortably on the edge of your chair with your feet firmly planted on the ground.

Interlock your hands behind your head and slowly inhale.

As you exhale, lift your chin towards the ceiling and spread your elbows out towards the side.

Hold the stretch for 15-20 seconds while breathing deeply.

Gently come back to the starting position and repeat the stretch 3-5 times.

Take care not to strain your neck or back while doing the exercise and avoid extending your elbows beyond your comfort zone. If you feel any discomfort, reduce the intensity of the stretch and try again.

REPS: 3-5

SETS: 1

How to Progress in Difficulty:

- Work your way up to 3 sets
- Use a towel: grab a towel and position it behind your upper back and hold it above your head with both hands. Use the towel to pull your upper back towards the back of the chair. Hold the stretch for 30 seconds and repeat it 3-5 times.
- Change the arm position: instead of interlocking your hands behind your head, try holding your arms out straight in front of you. This variation will stretch different muscles in your chest.

Inner Thigh Stretch

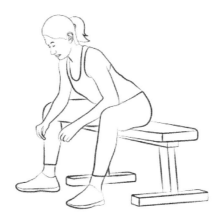

To begin the seated inner thigh stretch, sit in a straight-back chair with your feet flat on the ground.

Place your forearms on the inside of your knees and gently press your knees inward. Resist and push out with your arms. You should feel a stretch in your inner thighs.

Hold the stretch for 15-30 seconds and release.

REPS: 3-5

SETS: 1

How to Progress in Difficulty:

- Increase reps to 8-10
- Work your way up to 3 sets
- Hold for longer periods- up to 45 seconds
- do the same stretch, but with one foot lifted off the ground at a time
- Increase sets to 3

3. Shoulder Shrug

Sit on a chair with your back straight and your feet flat on the floor.

Hold a weight or a water bottle (or nothing!) in each hand and let your arms hang down by your sides. Slowly lift your shoulders towards your ears while keeping your arms straight and exhaling.

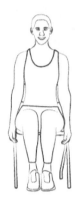 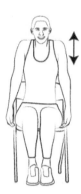

Hold the tension in your shoulders for 2-3 seconds, then lower your shoulders back down while inhaling. Push shoulders down and hold for 2-3 seconds.

REPS: 10-15

SETS: 1 start

How to Progress in Difficulty:

To make this exercise more difficult:

- Work your way up to 3 sets
- Add or increase the weights
- Hold the tension in your shoulders for a longer period
- Try alternating shoulder shrugs by lifting your left shoulder up while lowering your right shoulder and vice versa

4. Neck Turns

Start by sitting in a comfortable chair with your feet flat on the ground and hands resting on your lap.

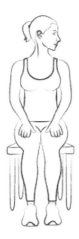 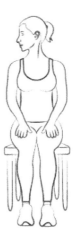

Begin by looking straight ahead and then slowly turn your head to look over your right shoulder. Hold the position for a few seconds and then return to the center.

Repeat on the left side.

REPS: 10 on each side

SETS: 1 to start

How to Progress in Difficulty:

- Increase reps to 15
- Work up to 3 sets
- Hold a small weight, such as a water bottle, with both hands and place it on your forehead. Then slowly turn your head to the right while keeping the weight in place. Hold for a few seconds and return to the center.

5. Seated Alternating Toe Touches

Sit on the edge of your chair, ideally with your feet flat on the floor and hip-width apart.

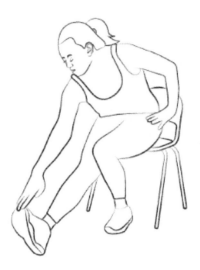

Lift your right leg off the floor and extend it forward, keeping it straight.

Reach your left hand towards your right toe, exhaling deeply as you do this. Try to touch your toe, but if you cannot reach, aim for your shin or ankle.

Hold this position for a second or two, then return your arm and leg to the starting position. Repeat the same movement on your left side, alternating between your right and left leg. Remember to maintain proper form throughout the exercise, keeping your back straight, and your core engaged as you reach for your toes.

REPS: 10-12 for each leg

SETS: 1 to start

How to Progress in Difficulty:

- Increase reps to 15

- Increase sets to 3
- Hold a weighted ball or a water bottle in your hands while performing the exercise to add resistance.
- Instead of touching your toes with your opposite hand, reach with both hands for your toes, working your abdominal muscles more intensely.
- Lift both legs off the ground and reach for your toes with both hands at the same time.

Cool Down

Now that we've completed our mobility exercises let's finish off with a quick cool-down session. Slowly shake out your arms and legs, and let your body relax. Breathe deeply in through your nose, hold for a few seconds, and then exhale.

Finally, give yourself a pat on the back and congratulate yourself for a job well done!

Notes on Today's Workout

How I Felt

_____

_____

_____

_____

What I Liked

_____

_____

_____

_____

What I Would Do Differently

_____

_____

_____

_____

Day 11

Arm Day

Warm Up

Welcome back for another day of chair exercises. Today, we will be working on Day 11 - another arm day. It's important for seniors to keep their arms strong and toned as it can help improve overall mobility and independence.

The Exercises

Before starting the exercises, let's start with a 5-minute warm-up. To begin, sit up tall in your chair with your feet planted on the ground and your hands on your knees.

Start by simply shrugging your shoulders up towards your ears, then release. Do this 10 times.

Next, roll your shoulders forwards 10 times, and then roll them backward 10 times. This helps to loosen up the muscles in your shoulders. Now, take your right hand and extend it straight out in front of you.

With your left hand, grab your right wrist and gently pull it towards your body until you feel a stretch in your arm. Hold this stretch for 10 seconds, and then switch arms. Repeat this 2 times on each side.

Bicep Curls

Start by sitting tall in a sturdy chair with your feet flat on the ground. Hold a weight in each hand, keeping your palms facing up and your elbows close to your sides. Begin with a weight that feels comfortable for you, such as 1-2 pounds.

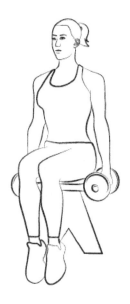 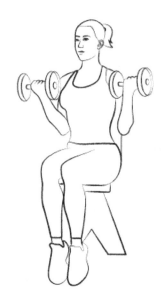

Slowly lift the weights towards your shoulders, keeping your elbows in place by your sides. Hold the contraction for a second or two, then slowly lower the weights back down to the starting position.

REPS: 10-12

SETS: 2

It's important to focus on using your biceps to lift the weights, not your shoulders or back.

How to Progress in Difficulty:

- Increase reps to 15
- Increase sets to 3
- Increase weight, gradually
- Add a pause at the top of the movement

Cross Body Jabs

Sit up straight and place your feet hip-width apart on the floor.

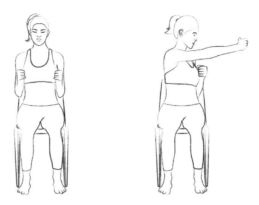

Make fists in front of your chest with your elbows bent. Tighten your core muscles and twist your torso to the right, punching your right arm across your body towards the left. Keep your left arm stationary.

Return to the starting position and repeat on the other side, twisting your torso to the left and punching with your left arm.

Continue alternating punches for 30-60 seconds, or until you feel fatigued.

SETS: start with 1

How to Progress in Difficulty:

As you get more skilled with this exercise, you can make it harder by doing any of the following:

- Increase the speed of your punches.
- Hold a small weight or resistance band in your hands.
- Add a leg lift with each punch, lifting the opposite foot off the floor as you twist.
- Try standing up and doing the exercise with or without hand weights.

3. Bow String Pull-Back

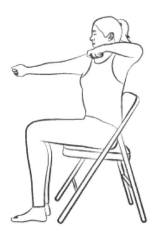

Sit on a sturdy and comfortable chair. Sit up tall with your feet flat on the floor and back straight. Engage your core muscles. Stretch your arms out straight in front of you, palms facing each other.

Slowly pull your right arm back as if you're pulling a bow string. As you do so, squeeze your shoulder blades together, hold for a few seconds, then release. Repeat using the left arm to pull.

Remember to breathe regularly throughout the exercise. The movement should be smooth and controlled.

REPS: 10-12

SETS: start with 2

How to Progress in Difficulty:

- Increase reps to 15
- Work your way up to 3 sets
- increase the intensity by adding weight to both hands

4. Triceps Extensions

Sit on your chair with your back straight and hold a weight with both hands behind your head.

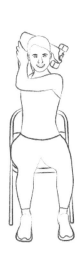 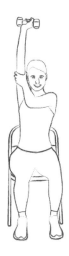

Keep your elbows close to your ears and extend your arms up to bring the dumbbell straight above your head.

Now slowly lower the dumbbell down to the nape of your neck while keeping your elbows close to your ears.

REPS: 8-10

SETS: 2

How to Progress in Difficulty:

- Increase reps to 15
- Work your way up to 3 sets
- Gradually increase the weight

5. Overhead Press

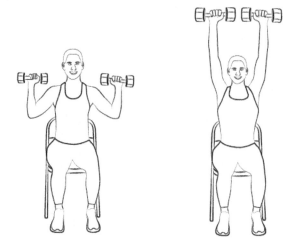

To start, sit on a chair with your back straight, and feet flat on the ground. Hold a lightweight dumbbell in each hand with palms facing forward.

Bend your elbows and raise your arms to shoulder level, with the elbows bent at a 90-degree angle.

Slowly straighten your arms, lifting the weights towards the ceiling, and take a deep breath. Bring the weights back down to shoulder level and exhale.

REPS: 10 (you may need to work up to this-that's OK!)

SETS: start with 1

How to Progress in Difficulty:

- Increase reps to 15 in each set
- Increase sets to 3- gradually
- Increase weight

Cool Down

Before wrapping up the workout, let's do a cool-down. Start by sitting up tall in your chair with your feet planted on the ground.

Take your right arm and bring it behind your head, using your left hand to gently push your elbow down. Hold this stretch for 10 seconds, then repeat on the other side.

Next, take your right arm across your chest, using your left hand to gently pull it across your body. Hold this stretch for 10 seconds and repeat on the other side.

Finally, take your right hand and place it on your left shoulder, using your left hand to gently push down on your elbow. Hold this stretch for 10 seconds, then repeat on the other side.

Notes on Today's Workout

How I Felt

_____

_____

_____

_____

What I Liked

_____

_____

_____

_____

What I Would Do Differently

_____

_____

_____

_____

Day 12

Leg Day

Welcome back! Today, we're focusing again on leg day - one of the most important parts of the body for seniors to exercise. As we age, our legs tend to weaken, leading to the loss of balance and increasing the risk of falls. However, with just a few simple chair exercises, you can strengthen your legs and improve your overall mobility and quality of life.

Warm Up

Start by sitting up straight in your chair with your feet flat on the ground and your hands on your thighs. Take a few deep breaths and gently roll your shoulders back and forth.

Next, lift your right leg and rotate your ankle clockwise and then counterclockwise, repeating with your left leg. Then, lift and lower each leg, keeping your knee straight.

The Exercises

Toe Taps

Sit towards the front of your chair with your feet flat on the floor.

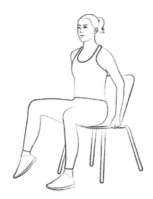

Keep your back straight and engage your core muscles. Lift your right foot off the floor and tap your toes lightly on the ground. Then, lift your left foot and tap your toes.

Continue alternating between your right and left foot, tapping your toes 30 seconds. It's important to keep your movements slow and controlled and avoid bouncing your feet off the floor.

REPS: 30 seconds

SETS: 1-2

How to Progress in Difficulty:

- Increase Reps to 60 seconds
- Work your way up to 3 sets
- Try moving your feet in a faster rhythm while still maintaining control.
- Instead of tapping your toes, try tapping your heels. Alternatively, you can tap your left foot twice before alternating to the right foot. This will help to engage different muscle groups.

- Add arm raises or punches while you tap your toes. This will help to engage your upper body as well.

Calf Raises

Sit on the edge of a sturdy chair with your feet flat on the ground.

Place your hands on your thighs or hold onto the sides of the seat.

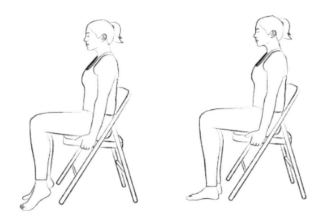

Slowly raise both of your heels, keeping your toes on the ground until you feel your calf muscle engaged.

Pause for 2-3 seconds, then slowly lower your heels back to the ground.

REPS: 10-12

SETS: start with one

How to Progress in Difficulty:

Increase reps to 15-20

- Work up to 3 sets
- Hold a lightweight, like a water bottle, in each hand while doing calf raises.

- Hold the top of the calf raise for an extra few seconds before lowering your heels.

Glute Squeezes

First, sit on a sturdy, non-slip chair with your feet planted firmly on the ground. Keep your back straight, shoulders relaxed, and hands resting on your thighs.

Next, tighten your glutes by squeezing your buttocks muscles. Hold for a count of 5, then release slowly. There are no pictures for this …but YOU"VE GOT THIS!

REPS: 5-10

Sets: 1 to start

How to Progress in Difficulty:

☒ Increase reps to 10-15

☒ Work up to 3 sets

☒ Increase the duration of each squeeze and release.

☒ Add resistance by placing a folded towel or cushion between your knees.

☒ Lift one foot slightly off the ground while squeezing with the opposite glute.

Ankle Circles

Sit on a chair with your back straight and your feet flat on the ground.

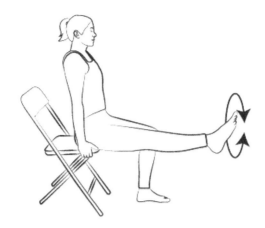

Lift your right foot off the ground and rotate your foot clockwise for 10-15 seconds (not the whole leg).

Rotate your foot counterclockwise for 10-15 seconds.

Repeat this with your left foot.

REPS: 10-15 seconds per foot

SETS: start with 2

How to Progress in Difficulty:

- Gradually increase the time you spend on each rotation until you can do 30 seconds each way.
- Increase sets to 3
- Try the exercise with your eyes closed. This is a great way to challenge your balance and improve stability.
- Add ankle weights.

5. Knee Extensions

Start by sitting upright in your chair with your back straight and your feet firmly planted on the ground.

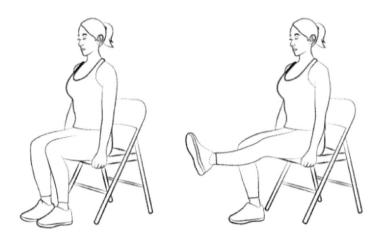

Slowly extend one leg out in front of you, keeping your foot flexed and your knee in line with your hip. Flex your foot forward as if you are pushing against a wall.

Hold the position for 2-3 seconds, then slowly lower your leg back down to the starting position.

Repeat the exercise with the other leg.

REPS: 8-12 on each leg

SETS: 1-2 to start

How to Progress in Difficulty:

To increase the difficulty of this exercise, try the following:

- Increase the number of repetitions: Gradually build up to 15-20 repetitions per leg.

- Increase sets to 3
- Add ankle weights: This will increase resistance and build strength.
- Hold a ball between your knees: This will engage your inner thigh muscles as well as your quadriceps.
- Slow down the movement: Moving more slowly will engage your muscles for longer and make the exercise more challenging.

Cool Down

Sit up straight in your chair with your feet flat on the ground. Cross your right ankle over your left knee and gently press down on your right knee until you feel a stretch in your right hip. Hold for 30 seconds, then repeat on the other side.

Notes on Today's Workout

How I Felt

_____

_____

_____

_____

What I Liked

_____

_____

_____

_____

What I Would Do Differently

_____

_____

_____

_____

Day 13

Core Day

Today is Day 13, which means we will be focusing on your core muscles. Having a strong core is essential for maintaining balance and stability, reducing the risk of falls, and improving your posture. As always, we will start with a warm-up and end with a cool-down, so grab a chair and let's get started!

Warm Up

Start by sitting up straight in your chair, with your feet flat on the floor and your hands on your thighs. Take a deep breath in, then exhale slowly while you tilt your pelvis forward and backward, flexing and extending your lower back. Repeat this movement 5-10 times, then sit back up straight.

Next, interlace your fingers and reach your arms overhead, stretching your entire body from your fingertips to your toes. Hold for a few seconds, then release and shake out your arms.

Finally, place your hands on your hips and rotate your torso to the right, then to the left. Repeat this movement a few times, focusing on the stretch in your oblique muscles.

The Exercises

Seated Alternating Toe Touches

Sit on the edge of your chair, ideally with your feet flat on the floor and hip-width apart.

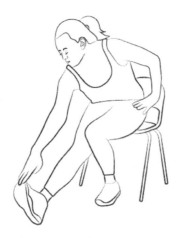

Lift your right leg off the floor and extend it forward, keeping it straight.

Reach your left hand towards your right toe, exhaling deeply as you do this. Try to touch your toe, but if you cannot reach, aim for your shin or ankle.

Hold this position for a second or two, then return your arm and leg to the starting position. Repeat the same movement on your left side, alternating between your right and left leg. Remember to maintain proper form throughout the exercise, keeping your back straight, and your core engaged as you reach for your toes.

REPS: 10-12 for each leg

SETS: 1 to start

How to Progress in Difficulty:

- Increase reps to 15
- Increase sets to 3
- Hold a weighted ball or a water bottle in your hands while performing the exercise to add resistance.

- Instead of touching your toes with your opposite hand, reach with both hands for your toes, working your abdominal muscles more intensely.

- Lift both legs off the ground and reach for your toes with both hands at the same time.

2 .Modified Push-Ups

To perform a modified push-up, sit on the edge of a chair and place your hands on either side of your hips, gripping the armrests.

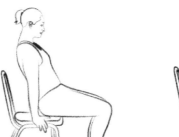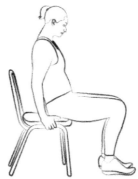

Keeping your back straight, lift your bottom off the chair and hold it for 10 seconds.

Then, lower it back down to the chair. It's important to engage your core muscles while performing this exercise. If you find the exercise challenging, you can start by doing the movement less intensely, such as gently lifting your bottom off the chair instead of holding it or even just lifting one cheek. You will gradually work your way up to the full movement.

REPS: 8-10

SETS: 1 to start

How to Progress in Difficulty:

- Increase reps to 12-15

- Increase sets to 3

- try lifting one leg off the ground at a time during the hold

- increase the holding time from 10 seconds to 20 seconds

3.March in Place

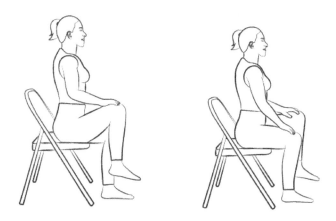

Sit up straight in your chair with your feet flat on the floor. Make sure your chair is stable and won't tip over. Keep your back straight and engage your core muscles.

Start by marching only your right leg up and down, as if you're marching in place. Keep the movement slow and controlled.

After 30 seconds, switch to your left leg and march for another 30 seconds. Repeat the cycle.

REPS: 1 30 second march on each side

SETS: start with 1

How to Progress in Difficulty:

- Increase to 2, then 3 sets
- Try raising your knees higher
- Add ankle weights
- Introduce hand weights while marching

4.Alternating Cross Body Crunch

Begin by sitting straight on a chair. Put your hands behind your head or grip the chair with both hands.

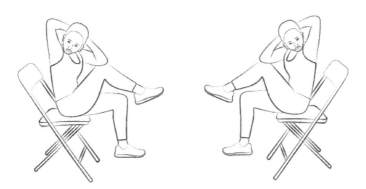

Lift your right knee and bring it towards your left elbow, twisting your torso to the right. Repeat on the other side: lift your left knee and bring it towards your right elbow while twisting to the left.

Do this in alternating fashion, as if you are pedaling a bicycle while crunching your sides.

REPS: 8-10 each side

SETS: start with 1

How to Progress in Difficulty:

- Increase reps to 12-15 each side

- Work up to 3 sets

- Hold a water bottle in each hand while executing the crunches for added resistance.

- Slow down the motion and hold each side crunch for 2-3 seconds before switching to the other side.

Side Stretch

Sit in a chair with your feet flat on the ground and your hands resting on your lap. Ensure that your chest is up, your shoulders are relaxed, and your spine is straight.

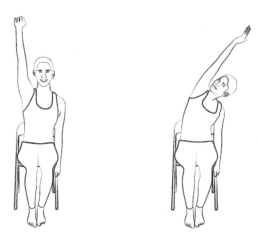

Place your right hand on the side of your chair and reach upwards with your left hand to stretch your left arm up over your head and bend to the right.

Hold the stretch for 20-30 seconds, inhaling and exhaling deeply.

Bring your left hand down to rest on your lap, then repeat the stretch on the opposite side, using your left hand on the side of the chair and your right arm reaching upwards.

REPS: 5 stretches on each side

SETS: 1 to start

How to Progress in Difficulty:

- Increase the number of repetitions you do per session.

- Work your way up to 3 sets

- Gradually increase the range of motion by stretching your arms further as you bend to the side.

- Alternate the seated side stretch with standing side stretches to increase the intensity of the exercise.

Cool Down

After you've finished your core exercises, it's important to cool down and stretch your muscles.

Sit up straight with your feet flat on the floor and your arms at your sides. Reach your left arm up and over your head, bending to the right and feeling the stretch along your left side. Hold for a few seconds before releasing and repeating on the other side.

Sit up straight with your feet flat on the floor and your hands on your thighs. Inhale and arch your back, lifting your chest towards the ceiling. Exhale and round your spine, tucking your chin to your chest. Repeat for a few breaths.

Notes on Today's Workout

How I Felt

_____

_____

_____

_____

What I Liked

_____

_____

_____

_____

What I Would Do Differently

_____

_____

_____

_____

Day 14

Full Body Day

On this fourteenth and final day of our exercise program, we will be focusing on a full body workout.

Warm Up

Start by sitting up straight in your chair, feet flat on the floor, and shoulders relaxed. Take a deep breath in, and as you exhale, roll your shoulders back and down. Repeat this shoulder roll a few times.

Next, place your hands on your thighs and lift one knee towards your chest. Hold for a few seconds before lowering your foot back to the ground. Alternate between your right and left leg for about 30 seconds.

Finally, extend your arms out to the sides and rotate your torso from side to side. This will warm up your core muscles and get your blood flowing.

The Exercises

Chest Stretch

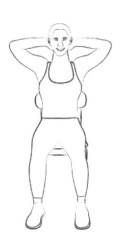

Begin by sitting comfortably on the edge of your chair with your feet firmly planted on the ground.

Interlock your hands behind your head and slowly inhale. As you exhale, lift your chin towards the ceiling and spread your elbows out towards the side.

Hold the stretch for 15-20 seconds while breathing deeply.

Gently come back to the starting position and repeat the stretch 3-5 times.

Take care not to strain your neck or back while doing the exercise and avoid extending your elbows beyond your comfort zone. If you feel any discomfort, reduce the intensity of the stretch and try again.

REPS: 3-5

SETS: 1

How to Progress in Difficulty:

- Work your way up to 3 sets
- Use a towel: grab a towel and position it behind your upper back and hold it above your head with both hands. Use the towel to pull your upper back towards the back of the chair. Hold the stretch for 30 seconds and repeat it 3-5 times.
- Change the arm position: instead of interlocking your hands behind your head, try holding your arms out straight in front of you. This variation will stretch different muscles in your chest.

2. Seated Jack

Sit up straight in your chair with your feet firmly planted on the ground.

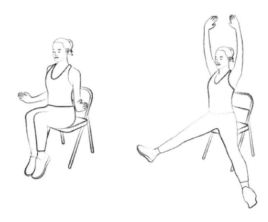

Place your hands on the armrests of your chair and begin moving feet in and out (as if you were doing a jumping jack motion with your lower body).

As you move, bring your hands overhead and clap them together at the top of the motion.

Keep your movements controlled and steady, making sure to engage your core muscles throughout the exercise.

REPS: Continue for 30 seconds

SETS: start with 1

How to Progress in Difficulty:

- Increase rep to 60 seconds
- Work your way up to 3 sets
- Increase the speed of movements
- Hold onto a weight

3. Heel Slides

Sit upright in a sturdy chair with your feet flat on the ground and your back straight.

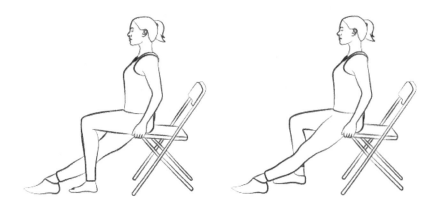

Slowly slide your right heel towards your buttocks, bending your knee as far as you comfortably can.

Hold the position for a few seconds, then slowly slide your heel back to the starting position.

Repeat on the other side, alternating between your left and right heel.

REPS: 15 per leg

SETS: start with 1

How to Progress in Difficulty:

- Work up to 3 sets
- You can make heel slides more challenging by wearing ankle weights, starting with 1 or 2 pounds and gradually increasing the weight.
- Alternate legs in a skating motion

4 . Front Shoulder Raises

To start, sit comfortably in a chair with your feet flat on the ground and your back straight.

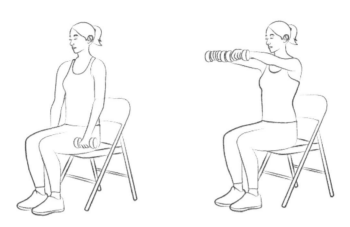

Hold a weight in each hand with your palms facing down and your arms extended down. (Its ok to not use any weights if that feels right to start with.)

Then, slowly raise your arms in front of you, keeping them straight and parallel to the ground. Stop when your arms are about shoulder level and hold for a few seconds before slowly lowering your arms back down to starting position.

REPS: 8-10

SETS: start with 2

How to Progress in Difficulty:

- Increase reps to 15 per set
- Increase sets to 3
- Increase weight (gradually)

5.Leg Circles

Begin by sitting upright in a chair with your back straight and your feet firmly planted on the floor. Make sure the chair is sturdy and won't move around. Place your hands on the sides of the chair for support.

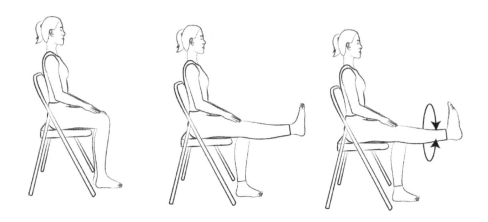

Lift one leg up, so your knee is at a 90-degree angle, parallel to the floor. Keep your foot flexed for stability.

Slowly rotate your leg in a circular motion, starting from your hip joint. Make sure to keep your back straight and your core engaged throughout the exercise. Complete the circle by bringing your leg down and back to its starting position.

REPS: 8-10/leg

SETS: 1 to start

How to Progress in Difficulty:

- Increase the number of repetitions to 15 gradually
- Increase the number of sets to 3
- Add ankle weights for more resistance
- Increase the size of the circular motion
- Alternate directions, working both clockwise and counterclockwise

Cool Down

After completing the full-body exercises, it's important to cool down your muscles. Start by slowing down your breathing and taking deep breaths in and out. Next, stretch your arms out in front of you and gently raise them up towards the ceiling. Hold for a few seconds before lowering your arms back down.

Finally, stretch your legs out in front of you and point your toes towards the ceiling. Reach towards your toes, stretching your hamstrings. Hold for 10-15 seconds before releasing.

Notes on Today's Workout

How I Felt

_____

_____

_____

_____

What I Liked

_____

_____

_____

_____

What I Would Do Differently

_____

_____

_____

_____

Conclusion

Congratulations on completing this series of chair exercises!

Hopefully, you've gained some valuable insight into the wide range of exercises you can do - and all from a chair, at that.

Not only are these exercises a great way to stay active, but they can help reduce the risk of injury and improve your overall well-being. These exercises provide benefits such as improved balance, increased strength and flexibility, better oxygenation of tissues, and improved overall health.

As another reminder, always consult with your doctor before beginning any new exercise program and keep them in the loop about your progress as you continue on your fitness journey.

There is no "one-size-fits-all" approach when it comes to health and fitness; what works for some people may not work for others. Your doctor will be able to provide the most accurate advice tailored to your individual needs.

If this book has helped you or someone you know discover chair exercises, we would love to hear from you! Please consider leaving us a review online so we can continue helping our senior community stay active and healthy.

Thank you for joining us!

Made in the USA
Las Vegas, NV
17 October 2023

79219888R00077